The 100 Powerful Prayers for Humor

Start With Self-Talk to Make Others Laugh Hysterically...

Toby Peterson

Copyright © 2016 PrayToTheWorld.com All Rights Reserved.

No part of this publication may be reproduced, distributed, or transmitted in any form or by any means, including photocopying, recording, or other electronic or mechanical methods, or by any information storage and retrieval system without the prior written permission of the publisher, except in the case of very brief quotations embodied in critical reviews and certain other noncommercial uses permitted by copyright law.

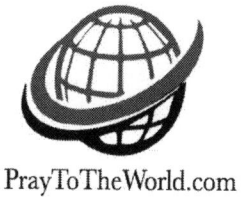

PrayToTheWorld.com

Do You Know **Exactly** How Prayer Changes Lives?

We'd like to give you a FREE copy of our book: Prayer Will Change Your Life, available only & exclusively at PrayToTheWorld.com.

Prayer Will Change Your Life gives you step-by-step actions on why you need to use the power of prayer in your daily life. It's also the precursor to all of PrayToTheWorld.com's Most Powerful Prayer Series.

This title is not available on Amazon, iBooks or Nook. It's only available at PrayToTheWorld.com.

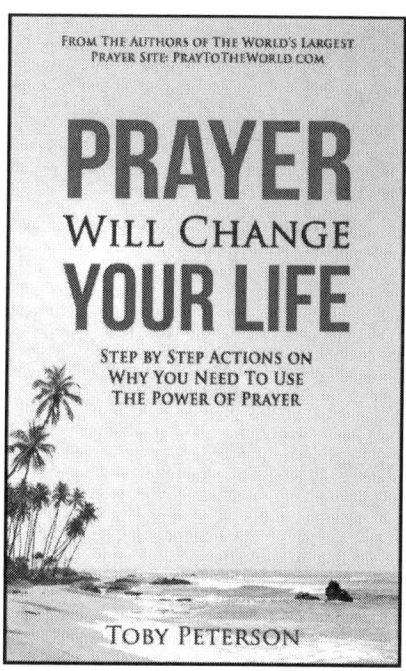

Table of Contents

Before You Start

Introduction .... *i*

The 100 Most Powerful Prayers for Humor 3

Bonus Books:

The 100 Most Powerful Prayers for Public speaking 27

The 100 Most Powerful Prayers for Happiness......... 51

Conclusion..75

Introduction

You are now taking the first steps to achieving fulfillment and happiness through God by becoming the architect of your own reality.

Imagine that with a few moments each day, you could begin the powerful transformation toward complete control of your own life and well being through prayer.

Because you can begin that powerful transformation with God, right now.

You will be able to release all fear and doubt simply because you know God gives you the power. You can utilize this simple, proven technique to regain the lost comforts of God's joy, love, and fulfillment in your life.

You have the ability to unlock God's full potential inside of yourself and achieve your ultimate goals. This is the age-old secret of the financial elite, world-class scholars, and Olympic champions. When you watch the Olympics you'll find one consistency in all of the champions. Each one closes their eyes to pray for a moment and clearly visualizes themselves completing the event flawlessly just before starting. And then, they win gold medals and become champions. These crisp visualizations are a way of prayer that history's most accomplished and fulfilled heroes have been using for centuries. That's merely one example of how the real power of prayer can help God to elevate you above any of life's challenges.

As you begin to attune yourself to God's positive energy around you it will become easier and easier to create the world you perceive.

Prayer isn't intended to make you delude yourself or simply throw a blanket over the negative aspects of your life. The intentions are to magnify your focus on the positive reality you desire and the endless possibility of God to help you make it so. Prayer will not force you to get up from your chair and magically start a multi-billion dollar business in a single day. But, prayer will help you take control of your motivation and release doubt, giving you the power to pave the steps in front of you as you stride confidently with God toward manifesting your goals.

You are now striding confidently with God toward manifesting your goals.

Many people lose themselves in the daily cycle of life and all of its stressing factors. As you mold these prayers into your psyche, you'll find that God will leave less and less room for the anxiety and fear that cripples so many people's well being. You will find the prayers here will help you find God's strength to carry on toward personal satisfaction despite life's troubles and anxieties.

God is now releasing you from a cycle of negative thinking and pessimism.

Many prayers in this book may stick with you or touch you in a very spiritual way. Please feel free to take them into your daily life and use them. There is no reason to stick rigidly to the use of any particular set of prayers, or to limit your use of them. Keep trying and find out what works for you. If it makes you feel positive and empowered, God is working wonders in your life.

These affirmations are for use everywhere. As you begin to use them, you will find yourself remembering certain ones in certain stressful situations. This is your consciousness learning to replace negative patterns with prayer. When you feel this begin to happen, don't worry! The tingling means it's working.

By utilizing prayer you are training your consciousness to work in tandem with God's natural flow of energy. This is how we are naturally designed to function as happy, healthy beings. Unfortunately, the complexity of the world has made it more difficult to find the natural creative harmony God placed inside each of us. Negative thinking goes against God's natural order of the universe and will unravel along with those who harbor it. Through prayer you will learn to be constantly over-filled with positive energies that soak into the world and the people around you.

If you want to see positive change now, you'll find the quickest path to fulfillment with prayer. There is no time to spend on loss, negativity, and defeat when you can be achieving tangible, historically proven results with minimum time and effort invested.

Consider the following your prescription for results:

1. Review the following list of prayers in full.

2. Pick Five to Ten prayers that powerfully resonate with you.

3. Repeat several times a day at different intervals. (Minimum Five times a day)

4. Use anything available to remind you during a busy day: a daily planner, phone alarm, etc.

5. Do this consistently for Ninety Days.

At the end of these ninety days, you will notice, without doubt, that less and less is happening to you in your life by default. Then you can repeat with the next subject that you wish to make powerful change in your life with.

Enjoy!

The 100 Most Powerful Prayers for Humor

I am created by God to humor people and make them happy...

I am God's chosen instrument of happiness, humor, and laughter...

I am happy and need to share this happiness with the Lord's people...

Thank you, Lord, for I have a lot of reasons to laugh and be happy about...

I am blessed with funny bones, wit, and decent humor...

I find making people laugh a natural instinct and a blessing from God...

I am blessed to be a natural optimist amidst my own sufferings...

I allow God to take over when times get rough but I still need to laugh...

Lord, help me remember funny and happy situations when I am surrounded by life's turbulences...

Jesus, help me to understand that You put me in a difficult situation for me to treasure my gift of humor...

Lord, let me be the lamp to light a gloomy place by making people laugh and forgetting their woes...

Allow me to obey Your command, oh God, to be a blessing to someone by making that person smile...

Lord, help me remain decent and grounded amidst my jokes and humor...

I am thankful for my gift of humor; the Lord has blessed me with more reasons to be happy...

I share humor and laughter and the Lord showers me with more than what I need...

I had nothing until the Lord gave me the gift of making people laugh...

Lord, show me where there is laughter and allow me to stay where there is gloom until it's gone...

My God, help me prove to everyone that every person is blessed with a reason to smile...

The Lord has blessed those who desire happiness and work hard to make people laugh and be merry...

I pray that everybody will find in their hearts the value of good humor today and always...

I am happy and when I am not, I am comforted with the thought that the Lord is just taking time to make me laugh...

God rewards me with a life full of humor and laughter...

I seize every opportunity that God gives me to make other people burst into laughter...

I am blessed with happiness, health, and wisdom from the Lord who sent me to make people laugh...

I will never get tired of finding reasons to smile or laugh about because the Lord strengthens me...

I always ask God to be with me so I won't be offensive when I crack jokes...

I will comfort people with my humor even when I am hurting because the Lord has instructed me to...

I am never short of humor; the Lord fills my cup...

I change tears to laughter and sadness to happiness through my jokes and prayers...

I am always happy because the Lord created me this way...

I pray whenever I am sad and then I am filled with humor and positivity...

I pray that with my sense of humor, the world will be a better place...

I truly believe that Jesus will not put me in a difficult situation that I can't handle with prayers and a dose of optimism and humor...

I am the best comedian with the Lord creating my spiels...

I channel my prayers of thanksgiving through happiness and laughter...

I will be a blessing of goodwill and laughter to my fellowmen...

I will scatter the seeds of happiness because the Lord wants me to...

Whenever I feel constrained and down, I pray and finally I am happy...

I am willing to make others happy because the merriment from my God is overflowing...

I lifted my gloom to the Lord and He has blessed me with high spirits...

I am blessed with a basket full of wit and humor and there is no room for sadness...

I am neither beautiful nor rich but God has given me humor and the ability to look at the bright side, which are more than enough...

I am joyfully serving the Lord and spreading His Words with my humor...

I am happy with the Lord at my side — nothing can pull me down...

I feel great to make people happy and serve the Lord in my little ways...

I have friends who are happy and when they are not, God uses me and my humorous side to cheer them up...

I will use my wit and humor to serve the Lord...

I pray that my little acts of kindness can make someone happy...

I believe that laughter is the sound of God's love and peace...

I thank the Lord for smiling moments after life's storms...

I keep thinking that my problems are Lord's reminders that comedians are allowed to cry, too...

I am laughing out as loud as I can in grateful acknowledgment of what the Lord has given me...

I will use my gift of gab and humor to remind people of God's promise to take us to a greener pasture...

The Lord strengthens me so I can help someone see the brighter side of life by opening her heart through her smile...

I hope that someday, everyone will find true happiness in serving Jesus...

I am praying that people find in their hearts a reason to smile constantly...

Jesus, I lift my burdens to You so I can find greater joy in making someone smile even when I'm in pain...

I will forever be grateful to my God for my high spirits and jolly personality...

I am always amazed by how the Lord blesses me with more laughing moments today than yesterday...

I have never stopped thanking the Lord for ability to share my gift of humor...

I disperse God's kindness through happiness and humor that radiate within me...

The Lord may have not given me material wealth but I am a billionaire if my laughter and wit have a price...

I don't know how I can serve the Lord without my sense of humor...

I am counting my blessings every day and make my heart content...

Thank you, Jesus, for making me find peace in making people laugh through clean entertainment...

I promise You, my Master, that I will never highlight another person's flaws to get people laughing...

Lord, help me spread good laughter and happy vibrations to change the world for the better...

Let me treasure, my Lord, the happiness that is evoked from my joke...

I serve You, God, by making people happy; let the outburst of laughter be that reward for me...

I have found joy and contentment in the Lord and with Him I will remain...

I would rather be blessed with little riches and abundant happiness and humor than be truly wealthy but lonely and sad...

I look for sunshine in summertime or for a rainbow after the rain that the Lord promises me...

Lord, let me treasure happy memories to look back on when good times are gone...

Lord, please be with me as I go through life's series of ups and downs and I thank You for the ups and rises...

I have faith that all bad things will be replaced by good things in God's time...

I imagine a world full of happy faces when people forget greed and hatred...

I allow God to give me reasons to be happy and funny...

I let go of my troubles and let God take the reigns — I will let His humor shine through...

I will share my blessings and humor to those who are in need...

I will remember that if I don't find true happiness today, the Lord will give me more tomorrows to look forward to...

I will seek to find humor in whatever life hurls my way as the Lord has commanded me...

I will follow my Lord's command and be happy...

I toss all my cares away and smile as the world laughs at me for my Lord is with me...

I am contented my Lord, to humor people who laugh at my jokes but never at me...

Oh Lord, I love to see happy tears and aching jaws from laughing too hard...

I am praying to you, oh Lord, bless me with the wisdom to crack a funny joke that would enlighten at least one soul...

I have found real happiness in the Lord who gave me this gift of wit and humor...

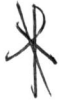 *My Lord, please remind me always that the key to contentment is counting happy moments first and paychecks last...*

I affirm that the Lord blesses me with a clean heart, a sound mind, and a good sense of humor...

I deserve to be happy because I share the Lord's blessings readily...

I am blessed knowing that a happy heart has pure intentions...

I pray that I will always be blessed with contentment and happiness starting today...

I asked for fun but the Good Lord has given me joy...

I pray that I will never blurt an insulting joke because happiness leaves no one injured...

I am grateful for my God-given sense of humor and countless opportunities to make someone smile...

Lord, please use me and my sense of humor to uplift someone's day...

I pray to God that if He ever stripped me off all blessings except one, my sense of humor will remain...

God, help me to always remember that my gift of good humor has its responsibilities, too...

I am blessed with wit and clean jokes that make someone smile...

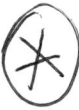 *My fulfillment is serving the Lord by making people happy...*

The 100 Most Powerful Prayers for Public Speaking

I am blessed to be a great public speaker...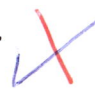

I am blessed to be able to make people focus on me when I talk to them...

I will speak with confidence and strength from God...

I speak clearly and concisely with confidence from God...

I find it easy to convey my thoughts and prayers in the simplest way possible...

I inspire people with my faith and my words...

I have been blessed with an expansive vocabulary at my disposal... ✗

I pray to command the attention of an audience... ✓

I am created by God as an interesting person to listen to... ✗

I have been blessed with a charming speaking voice... ✓

I speak with poise and eloquence from God... ✗

I am good looking and people notice me radiating God's grace... ✗

I am blessed to be a respected and admired speaker... ✓

I have been gifted by God with a welcoming voice and people love to listen to me...

I always smile and speak confidently to show God's grace... ✗

I am calm and relaxed in front of large groups because God is with me...

I am created to be a highly influential and charismatic person...

I find it easy to influence people that I speak to from God...

I am always able to make a convincing argument for God...

I speak God's truth from the bottom of my heart...

I find Influencing and persuading others toward God comes naturally to me...

I am letting God make me more articulate and influential every day...

I have been blessed by God and deserve all of my influential ability...

I enjoy being able to influence and persuade others for God...

I have been blessed with a convincing smile and personality...

I let God help me clearly understand what I am speaking about...

I get a thrill from speaking to large groups about God...

I am driven to share God's message with all the people I can...

I let God own the stage when I step onto it...

I am blessed by God to be an amazing communicator...

I am blessed to feel at home on a stage in front of people...

I let God make me compelling to every person in the group I am speaking to...

I inspire others to become capable public speakers and better Christians...

I let God make me more than ready to deliver my words...

I am able to let God give me the words I need when I open my mouth...

I feel passionate and driven when I speak about God...

I deserve every opportunity God gives me to speak...

I am blessed to be a celebrated public speaker...

I feel more relaxed and calm when I am speaking to people about God...

I radiate God's confidence from the stage...

I make a positive contribution to God's world every time I speak...

I feel completely at peace with God while I speak to people...

I have a powerful and magnetic presence from God...

I have been blessed with a naturally strong and commanding voice...

I have been blessed with an extensive vocabulary that I can draw from instantly...

I always let God give me the strength to speak clearly and loudly, projecting my voice over my audience...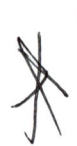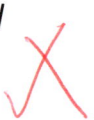

I am blessed to easily memorize speeches and monologues...

I am well groomed to project God's glory so that people enjoy looking at me while I speak...

I will let God help me keep the attention of every person I speak to...

I let God put me in control of every conversation I am having...

I let God help me deliver my words in a way the carries weight and conveys emotion...

I am blessed to be able to show people new ideas and concepts in an understandable way...

I am able to communicate about God with people from all walks of life...

I feel excited about God each time I take center stage...

I am always prepared by God to give a speech...

I am blessed to be able to rouse a group to action with a carefully engineered speech...

I am able to use my faith to help encourage others to see reason...

I let God make me a better speaker every time I do it... ✗

I let God help me leave a memorable mark on each person who hears me speak...

I am letting God help me foster a lucrative career as a public speaker... ✓

I am blessed to be clever, smart, and funny...

I let God give me eloquent responses to questions every time...

I have been put in God's world to speak to others...

I am able to turn enemies into friends using God's words...

I use my speaking ability to make God's world a better place...

I have God's unshakable confidence when I walk onto the stage...

I have been blessed with a constantly expanding vocabulary...

I let God teach me every chance I get to speak in public...

I am created by God to be a qualified and highly skilled orator...

I have been blessed with a total mastery of the spoken English language...

I have a spring of God's limitless charismatic energy flowing inside me...

I let God make me brave enough to speak to people who disagree with me...

I am created by God to be able to change people's minds easily...

I leave a lasting impact for God on the people who hear me speak...

I let God help me deliver speeches as if they are thought up on the spot...

I am blessed to be able to think of witty jokes easily on the spot...

I am blessed to naturally draw the focus of a group with the sound of my voice...

I accompany my confident voice with matching posture and mannerisms that God gave me...

I am blessed to be able to easily simplify complicated concepts...

I speak with God's clarity and precision...

I change lives for God each time I speak to a group...

I have been blessed with an energetic and outgoing personality...

I never experience stage fright, only excitement from God...

I am blessed to be remembered by each person who hears me speak...

I know how to appeal to many of God's different people...

I am able to let God make benign subjects appear exciting and interesting...

I am proud of the ability God gave me to speak in public...

I was created to speak to people and affect their lives...

I am blessed to make a fantastic living as a public speaker...

I enjoy letting God show me new subjects to talk about...

I am grateful for the ability God gave me to influence people...

I am blessed to be able to quickly dismiss interruptions and move on with my speaking...

I am able to use as few words as possible to let God help me convey complicated ideas...

I never turn down an opportunity God gives me to share my words with others...

I let God make other people want to understand what I'm trying to convey...

I have an ability to speak that is a gift from God that puts me on a higher level than most...

I have a strong spiritual presence that radiates with magnetic energy...

I am filled with a deep satisfaction from God after speaking to a large group...

I derive my life's greatest thrill and joy from the chances God gives me to speak in public...

I am blessed to be an influential, capable, and confident public speaker...

The 100 Most Powerful Prayers for Happiness

I am letting God teach me to become a more joyful person every day...

I will amplify the happiness God brings into my life...

I have been blessed with a wonderfully rewarding and contented life...

I am thankful for the abundant joy God put in my life...

I find new ways to be a happier person with each passing moment God gives me...

I always find something God placed in my life that I can be happy about...

I choose to and deserve to be happy the way God made me...

I have made the decision to live the life God gave me in a state of total joy...

I will share God's abundant joy with everyone around me...

I am living a life that is completely immersed in God's happiness...

I share God's joy with others and receive it back in multitudes...

I am in charge of how I feel and I choose to be happy with God...

I am brimming with God's joyful energy...

I am lifted up above negative thinking by God's grace...

I keep positive thoughts that brighten the days God gives me...

I have been blessed with a consistently positive outlook…

I will keep a positive attitude to help spread the happiness God gives me…

I nurture my cheerful attitude with prayer throughout the day…

I feel every cell in my body resonate with God's joy…

I find new things to be happy about with each day God gives me…

I am living a life filled with God's sunshine and positive vibrations...

I smile often to activate my brain's God given feel-good response...

I am blessed to maintain a sense of humor and laugh often...

I always set aside time to experience happiness with God...

I am living life as a peaceful and joyful being of God...

I radiate God's happiness and enjoy life to the fullest...

I will always let God show me a reason to smile...

I will only entertain joyful thinking and prayer...

I am free to experience all of the joy God has to offer...

I make each day the happiest day that God gave me...

I am the personification of happiness and God's love...

I stay merry and carefree all the time through prayer...

I bring the gift of God's happiness to everyone I meet...

I am always happy to be who God made me...

I radiate God's joy regardless of circumstances around me...

I am committed to being as happy as possible through prayer...

I am happy and at peace with the world God created...

I enjoy laughing and I'm blessed to do it often...

I am able to find happiness in every moment God gives me...

I make my good cheer come from within by using prayer...

I practice happiness through prayer as a habit...

I know what makes me happy and I seek it out with God's help...

I use laughter and prayer to release tension and stress...

I am blessed to live a life of pure and exhilarating joy...

I lighten any atmosphere with the great sense of humor God gave me...

I will follow my faith and happiness where it takes me...

I love to be smiling all the time because God is with me...

I allow myself to experience happiness in every moment of the life God gave me...

I leave no room for sadness in my life because God is with me...

I think happy thoughts and speak happy words while I pray...

I have an inner happiness from God that grows every day...

I will let my happiness multiply and be abundant with prayer...

I have happiness in my life because I pray for it...

I am living a life that spreads God's joy into the world...

I have the power to make God's joy expand and grow...

I am blessed to be living a remarkably happy and rewarding life...

I have everything I need from God to live a perfectly happy life...

I will make each day a testament to God's love and the joy I feel...

I will always give thanks for all the happiness that God gives me...

I am eternally grateful to God for the joyful experience that I am living...

I have more reasons to be happy with every minute that God gives me...

I make the conscious choice to live a life of happiness with God...

I have a joy that comes from God...

I am happy because God wants me to be...

I find new reasons for happiness because I expect God to show them to me...

I will take time to nurture and feed the happiness God gives me...

I will maintain a positive outlook on what God will bring me next...

I am very pleased with where God has taken my life...

I like the person I am and the person God is making me...

I am letting every cell in my body be washed over with God's happiness...

I have a joyful light from God flowing inside of me...

I remember to smile because it feels good and reminds me of God...

I have a life that is immersed in positive thoughts and prayers...

I will set aside time each day to focus on my prayers and happiness...

I have a life of total happiness and love from God...

I am proud of the way I live the life God gave me...

I share God's happiness with others when we talk...

I will let go of my tension and stress to make room for more of God's joy...

I have a bottomless spring of God's joyful energy inside of me...

I have made a personal commitment to God and my own happiness...

I am lucky to have God's gift of a joy-filled life...

I have a talent for making God's happiness contagious...

I will not limit the happiness God can give me...

I celebrate the joyful life God gave me just by living it...

I can choose to let God make me happy...

I am always content with the life God gave me...

I easily cast aside doubt and sadness through prayer...

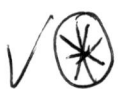

I make God and my own happiness my first priority...

I will appreciate each opportunity God gives me to feel joy...

I seize each chance God gives me to feel good and cherish it...

I love my life and the things that God has placed in it...

I feel good about who God made me and what I do...

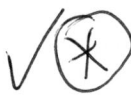

I am immune to negativity because God is with me...

I cannot be brought down by negative people because God is with me...

I am bathing in God's universal happiness...

I look forward to a future with even more of God's joy in store...

I use laughter to spread God's joy to other people in my life...

I love myself and the life God gave me...

I like looking forward to a wonderful future walking with God...

I am an unstoppable powerhouse of good vibrations and joy from God...

Thank You!

I want to sincerely thank you for reading this book!

Let me finish though by saying the work isn't done here. These must be put to use repetitively, and on a daily basis to see changes in your life.

Remember to follow the ninety-day plan outlined in the introduction to maximize your results.

Can I ask you for a very quick favor? Can you leave a review on our Amazon.com detail page to tell us about your progress and how you enjoyed the book?

We take the time to go over each review personally, and your feedback in invaluable to us as writers, and others that wish to see the same change in their lives as you:)

Thank You!

Printed in Great Britain
by Amazon